The Entire Body Reset for Adults:

This weight loss plan can help you achieve optimal health, a flat belly, and a body you love throughout midlife and beyond.

By

Clark K. Keen

1

TABLE OF CONTENTS

Introduction

It seems like a new trendy weight-loss diet presents itself whenever you walk out. These diets force you to restrict entire food groups or dramatically reduce the quantity of calories you consume, which might leave you feeling hungry and unsatisfied. Many people are unable to maintain their weight on these severe crash diets, which is why over 70% of Americans are either overweight or obese.

Celebrity trainer Harley Pasternak, who has worked with Hollywood elite such as Kim Kardashian, Rihana, and Natalie Portman, came up with the idea for the diet plan known as The Body Reset Diet after realizing how impossible it is to adhere to most diets. A smoothie-focused program that involves low-intensity activity is included in this diet plan, which lasts for fifteen days.

A little while after Jessica Simpson claimed that she had shed one hundred pounds, the diet instantly gained popularity through a partnership with Pastenak and adherence to the recommendations offered in his book, within six months.

The entire Body's Reset for Adults presents shocking new evidence about the power of "protein timing" for people who are in the middle of their lives.

This research disproves the current government guidelines, disproves the myth that slowing metabolisms and "inevitable" weight gain are inevitable, and alters how people in their mid-40s and older should think about food.

The Entire Body Reset for Adults provides a straightforward and motivational explanation of the age-related changes that occur in our bodies, as well as how adjusting our diet to accommodate these changes can cause us to respond to physical activity as if we were twenty to thirty years younger.

Diet phases, meal windows, calorie restriction, and other trendy gimmicks are not utilized in The Complete Body Reboot, which was developed by the American Association of Retired Persons (AARP), examined by a panel consisting of more than one hundred AARP employees, and authorized by an international board consisting of doctors, nutritionists, and fitness professionals.

The six straightforward secrets and scores of recipes that are included in it are simple to understand and were developed for actual people who live in the real world.

There is even a dining guide that demonstrates how to maintain compliance with this program in well-known places such as Olive Garden, Starbucks, and McDonald's. In addition to that, it is effective!

Chapter 1

What is the entire body reset?

Body reset can relate to several things, including diet and medical therapy. The body-reset diet is a diet plan that claims to reboot your metabolism and help you more efficiently burn calories by avoiding harmful foods, focusing on low-calorie, plant-based smoothies and other foods, and combining light exercise like walking.

On the other hand, a full-body reset is a medical treatment that sets up every area of your system to have a healthy response to food, sleep, exercise, and emotional triggers through doctor-prescribed medicine and lifestyle.

The body-reset diet is supposed to be just that: an abrupt reset to how you are eating by eliminating all solid foods and replacing them with nutritious, low-calorie, plant-based smoothies.

The "Body Reset" combines the "Resilience Boost" and "Gut Wellness Cleanse" courses into one comprehensive program. The Body Reset Plan says it would help you "eat more, exercise less" and still lose weight. The diet is geared primarily at people who have already tried several approaches to losing weight without success.

The Body Reset diet might promote some speedy weight loss, thanks to its low starting calorie allotment. It also promotes a realistic fitness plan. However, the short-term diet is unlikely to contribute to sustainable weight loss.

Harley Pasternak, a specialist in exercise physiology and nutritional sciences, created the Body Reset diet in 2013. During the next fifteen days, if you adhere to a plant-based diet that is low in calories and consists primarily of smoothies, you will be able to educate your body to use energy more efficiently and burn calories more quickly, even while you are sleeping.

1. A brief recap

As a result of the fact that nutrition is constantly changing, it can be difficult to follow a book like this from a particular date.

Even though the fundamentals of this plan, which include eating at regular intervals and maintaining a balanced diet, remain unchanged, if you do decide to give it a shot, you should opt for more modern versions of foods that fall into specific categories.

For example, if you consume dairy products, you should choose grass-fed, pasture-raised whole eggs. If you are an egg eater, you should choose pasture-raised whole eggs.

It is also a good idea to think about giving up beef, increasing the amount of seafood you consume, and increasing the number of meals that are plant-based. Finally, it's unknown how much weight you might lose in 15 days on this plan—or even how much weight you'll lose in six months, like Simpson.

Nevertheless, one thing is certain: losing weight and keeping it off does entail finding a method you can genuinely stick with and one that makes you feel well both physically and mentally. Whether that's this exact approach or your adaptation, in the long run, healthy, sane, and sustainable always wins out over fast and furious.

2. How does a body-reset diet work?

The Body Reset Diet claims to reboot your metabolism and help you more efficiently burn calories by avoiding harmful foods, focusing on low-calorie, plant-based smoothies and other foods, and combining light exercise like walking. This 15-day routine allows some flexibility in the foods you can choose but requires you to replace some meals with smoothies.

The very concept of trying to lose obesity is overwhelming for most, in large part due to the terrible goodbyes we may have to say to our favorite meals or the doubt that our new waistline will be sustainable.

These reasons probably account for the fact that fewer Americans than ever before are making an effort to lose weight. However, in this age of never-ending diet fads, the Body Reset plan offers a seductive new alternative: a low-exercise, smoothie-based 15-day cleanse that promises to help followers lose extra weight while maintaining it off.

Celebrity fitness expert and founder of the 5-Factors program, Harley Pasternak, who wanted to keep dieting easy, created the smoothie-based Body Reset program.

The idea behind the liquid diet, which was favored by Rihanna and Kim Kardashian, was to combine delicious cuisine in moderation with lots of movement and water consumption throughout the day. Except for solid meals as normal, liquid meals appear to spare the body nothing because they contain sufficient amounts of every food category.

Though you might be thinking, "Sign me up" at the idea of enjoying cocktails every day, there are a few things you should know before pulling out your food processor.

Similar to other short-term programs, such as the South Beach Diet or Inclusion30, Body Reset is divided into three five-day phases.

While the focus of each section is on various meal formats, smoothies all come from the same food source. Convenience is the main goal when creating a smoothie-based diet, according to Pasternak. It transports a variety of chemicals.

He does, however, guarantee that each smoothie has "comparable nutritional significance, fiber, protein, and healthy fats," despite variations in micronutrient content.

3. Fantastic! Will You Lose Weight After Adopting These Body Reset Dietary Practices?

The succinct reply is accurate. If you exercise regularly and watch what you eat, you should lose some weight. It's crucial to understand, though, that this is a temporary solution. "I don't think eating in any way for 15 days would have a lasting effect," contends Kelly Kennedy, RD, a specialty dietician for Daily Living.

While some people may find that going on a strict diet helps them lose weight quickly, Kennedy cautions that these drinks, which seem simple at first, could "be somewhat uninteresting" and advises giving them up.

4. Why Body Reset Should Be Used with Caution in People with Diabetic and Heart Conditions

Kennedy cautions anyone thinking about Body Reset who has heart problems or diabetes to approach it cautiously. Because of its high glucose content, the lunchtime "red" smoothie, also known as a fruit smoothie, can cause blood sugar levels to spike. Additionally, because it doesn't contain whole grains, it can be harmful to those who have heart disease.

U.S. News & World Report withdrew the Body Reset diet from its yearly list of diet reviews and rankings for a variety of reasons, including the fact that its panel no longer regarded the diet as a "viable eating plan."

Kennedy argues that drastically restricting whole grains eliminates one of the primary food groups that are advised for balance and to reduce "bad" LDL cholesterol, both of which are critical for heart health.

Kennedy recommends the DASH diet or the Mediterranean diet for a more well-rounded eating plan. "It's exactly the same diet I'd recommend for someone without diabetes," she says. "My two favorites are the DASH and Mediterranean diets because they're so well-balanced and emphasize obtaining your nutrients from whole foods.

5. How to Start the Body Reset Diet and What to Do Next

Ultimately, the best course of action is to consult your physician before making significant dietary changes. If you have heart disease or diabetes, you may want to reconsider following the strategy. Kennedy states that before doing something so drastic, "anyone with a pre-existing condition, really anyone in general, should be talking to their doctor."

13

Most important to understand is that Body Reset is aimed at quick, but not necessarily sustained, weight loss and relies on you to continue the lifestyle that it advocates even after the 15-day program is finished.

Chapter 2

The inside narrative of your stomach.

Your stomach, intestines, and colon are all part of your digestive system, which is known as your gut. It eliminates trash and breaks down and absorbs nutrients from food. There is no precise definition of gut health, and it can signify something to researchers, medical professionals, and the community.

Behind the screen of mystery, our stomach is responsible for bringing our body into operating condition. As it breaks down the foods we eat, our stomach absorbs nutrients that support our body's activities, from energy production to hormone balance, skin health to mental wellness, and even toxin and waste removal.

Over 70% of the immune system is housed in the gut, so making sure our digestive system is in tip-top shape can be crucial to resolving many of our body ailments. However, how do we transform our gut sensations into health solutions?

Your gut may not be a literal voice, but its functions communicate in a type of code. From utter silence to hunger grumbles and potty habits, receive insight into what is going on within.

We have all heard the phrase "trust your gut," and for good reason. The gut, and more crucially, the good bacteria residing inside it, are key participants in what makes our bodies function at their best. "What we're talking about is all these germs.

Normally, we speak more to the bacteria in the gut, but there are many different microorganisms. There's a whole bunch of these small cells down in our GI tract (gastrointestinal tract) that play a significant role in our health," she said.

"We have 10 times more cells in the gut than we do in any other area of our body," she added, and she highlighted various studies and scientific results, like the National Institutes of Health Human Microbiome Project. The goal is to prioritize this as a fundamental foundation for achieving optimal overall well-being.

1. What is abdominal fat?

Conditions that influence the metabolism of fat, the storage of fats, or other associated processes. The type of fat that gathers in your belly is called visceral fat. It is placed further inside your belly, encircling your internal organs. Visceral fat is significantly connected to greater resistance to the hormone insulin, which regulates your blood sugar levels.

 Over time, insulin resistance may lead to high blood sugar levels and the development of type 2 diabetes. Visceral fat also leads to systemic inflammation, which may enhance your illness risk.

It is crucial to know that carrying some fat in your belly is normal and serves to protect and insulate your body. However, having too much belly fat may affect your health and raise your risk of developing certain chronic conditions.

There are several healthy ways to remove excess belly fat, including increasing your consumption of nutrient-dense foods, getting enough sleep, and moving your body more.

There's not as much fat in your belly as there is throughout the rest of your body. There are two primary types of belly fat: one is found under your skin, and the other is found deeper inside your abdomen, around your internal organs. Subcutaneous fat and visceral adipose tissue (VAT)

2. The two forms of abdominal fat

(a) Subcutaneous fat

Subcutaneous fat, or subcutaneous adipose tissue (SAT), is the fat that is found under your skin. Subcutaneous fat is soft, and it is the fat you perceive as "jiggling" on your abdomen. In general, women have bigger amounts of subcutaneous fat than men.

Unlike the fat that is located deeper in the abdominal cavity, subcutaneous fat is not as strongly associated with a higher risk of illness.

However, having too much body fat in general, including total belly fat may increase your chance of acquiring several chronic conditions, such as type 2 diabetes, heart disease, and some malignancies. Contrarily, keeping healthy amounts of belly fat and overall body fat may help minimize your risk of acquiring a chronic disease.

(b) Visceral adipose tissue (VAT)

Visceral adipose tissue (VAT), or visceral belly fat, is the fat that surrounds internal organs like your kidneys, liver, and pancreas; therefore, it is much deeper in your abdomen than subcutaneous fat. This is usually referred to as "harmful" belly fat.

Compared with subcutaneous fat, visceral fat is substantially more metabolically active. This form of fat has more cells, blood vessels, and nerves than subcutaneous fat.

Visceral fat is significantly connected to greater resistance to the hormone insulin, which regulates your blood sugar levels. Over time, insulin resistance may lead to high blood sugar levels and the development of type 2 diabetes. Visceral fat also contributes to systemic inflammation, which may enhance your illness risk.

Men are more likely to build visceral fat than women, which is why men are more likely to have an "apple-shaped" figure as belly fat increases. On the other hand, women are more likely to gain excess fat in the lower body, resulting in a "pear" appearance.

Interestingly, body fat distribution changes with aging. For example, although premenopausal women have larger levels of subcutaneous belly fat, postmenopausal women tend to have higher levels of visceral fat, which contributes to an increased risk of metabolic disease.

Also, visceral fat tends to be larger in people of European heritage compared with people of other ethnicities.

3. Where does abdominal fat come from?

There are various reasons why people accumulate belly fat, including poor diet, lack of exercise, and stress. Improving nutrition, boosting activity, and making other lifestyle adjustments can help people lose belly fat.

A poor diet can induce belly fat. When a person consumes more calories than they expend for a while, it can cause weight gain and an increase in fat storage.

As a result, diets that contain a lot of high-calorie but low-nutritional meals can raise a person's risk of weight gain and belly fat levels.

The second crucial aspect of the energy in, energy out equation is a person's physical activity levels. A lack of physical exercise is a primary risk factor for obesity and a rise in body fat percentage. Increasing weight and physical inactivity might also make it tougher for a person to start exercising. When a person burns fewer calories through activity than they ingest, the body stores this surplus as fat.

A steroid hormone known as cortisol helps the body control and deal with stress. When a person is in a risky or high-pressure scenario, their body releases cortisol, altering their metabolism.

People often look for food for comfort when they feel worried. Cortisol enables those surplus calories to linger around the abdomen and other bodily locations for later utilization.

Chapter 3

A Day body reset

The Body Reset Diet is broken into three phases, each of which lasts 5 days and follows a precise diet plan comprised of smoothies, snacks, and solid meals.

- **Phase 1: Replace** breakfast, lunch, and dinner with smoothies and have two snacks per day. For physical activity, walk at least 10,000 steps each day.

- **Phase 2: Replace** 2 meals with smoothies, eat 1 full dinner, and have 2 snacks each day. For physical activity, walk 10,000 steps each day and complete 5 minutes of weight training utilizing 4 different exercises on 3 of the days.

- **Phase 3: Replace** 1 meal with a smoothie and eat 2 reduced-calorie meals and 2 snacks each day.
- For physical activity, walk 10,000 steps and conduct 5 minutes of weight training utilizing 4 different exercises every day.

After the diet is standard for 15 days, you're intended to follow the food plan specified in Phase 3 with one addition: twice-weekly "free meals" that allow you to eat or drink anything you want. These are included as a reward and a means to avoid feelings of deprivation.

Pasternak believes that repeatedly limiting yourself to your favorite foods may lead to binge eating. After the first 15 days, there is no formal endpoint to the diet for weight loss or maintenance. According to Pasternak, the routine and habits you have acquired in the first 15 days are supposed to be followed for a lifetime.

1. How to reset your entire body, with exercise and food

A diet and fitness routine can help you make the most of the body your genetics have given you. While you cannot change a lanky, lean frame into an hourglass, working out and eating healthily helps you lose weight, increase muscle, and feel more energetic.

Changing your body composition by increasing muscle and decreasing fat also enhances your stamina and makes you look firmer and more sculpted.

The amount of reshaping you can do depends on your current physique, how long you have to devote to the process, and your level of devotion.

Before putting on a diet and fitness plan, identify what reshaping means to you. You may desire to lower your size, get more toned and fit-looking, build up, or maybe even get thin enough to reveal a six-pack.

The first step in reducing fat and becoming stronger involves dietary and exercise commitment, but reaching the point of looking fitness-model thin takes substantial sacrifices and extra hard work. The larger the alteration you desire, the more behaviors you'll need to change. The extent to which you intend to reshape your physique impacts your diet and workout strategy.

For example, if you're an overweight man with an unhealthy body fat level of 23 percent or a woman with 32 percent, you'll modify your form by reducing the amount of fat consume.

The ideal amount of body fat for a guy is 18 percent, whereas for a woman it should be 25 percent. This entails decreasing calories, exercising several days per week, and giving up some indulgences, but you might find it a feasible approach.

If, however, you are already a relatively slim man who wants to reduce from 18 percent body fat to 14 percent

On the other hand, a relatively lean woman who wants to reduce from 25 percent to 20 percent, you'll need to commit to virtually daily workouts and forgo snacks most of the time.

Chapter 4

The six fundamental keys to optimal health

A new year. It is a fresh start and a time when many of us promise to make changes for the better. Unfortunately, for most of us, those pledges are forgotten a few weeks after they are made. That is typically because they are a bit too lofty and possibly too hard to maintain. The secret to establishing resolutions that stick is to make them simple.

A few little modifications can make a tremendous difference in your health. These six easy strategies for greater health are explained in the following paragraphs.

1. **Shake off the salt.** Decrease the quantity of salt you eat. Whole foods and plant-based foods are best. They are beneficial for you and can help you decrease your blood pressure.

   Try to make more food at home, and stay away from prepared goods and fast food. And if you can, avoid adding more salt to your diet.

2. **Lose a little.** Lose weight by lowering calories and eating complete foods and plants. Even shedding 10 pounds can make a major difference in your health and how you feel.

And any weight-loss regimen includes some activity. It boosts your probability of losing weight, your cardiovascular health, and your sense of well-being. Start by walking little distances, and expand on that every few days, just a little at a time.

3. **Partner with your provider.** Establish (or re-establish) a relationship with a primary care physician. They're the ones who should know you best—about your health history, your life, and its obstacles, and what precise screening checks you need at the major milestones in your life.

   They can provide you with methods that can help you get healthier and minimize your risk for problems like heart disease, diabetes, and stroke.

4. **Be smoke-free.** It is one of the most crucial things you can do. Smoking is the largest cause of preventable mortality and disease around the globe.

   Not being reliant on tobacco will make you healthier, and studies have proven it can make you happier. Consider calling the New York State Smokers' Quitline at 1-866-NY-QUITS or NYsmokefree.com.

The program gives plenty of information and services available to help you quit, including options such as nicotine replacement products.

5. **Ease up a bit.** Attempt to lessen your stress. It's a part of life for everyone, but be sure you are taking precautions to limit its impact. Identify some issue areas and explore what modifications might assist. Make time for yourself, even for a few minutes during a busy day. It may be as simple as slipping away for a quick cup of coffee. Perhaps consider meditation. There are mobile apps that can get you started.

6. **Don't skimp on sleep.** Adequate shut-eye permits us to better learn as we proceed through our day. It helps our memory. And it assists with both stress relief and weight gain (yes, there is a correlation between both of these and lack of sleep)

For adults, this means getting between seven and nine hours each night. Kids and teens need even more. It's a good idea to try and go to bed and get up at the same time each day, regardless of whether it's a work day, a weekend, or you're on vacation. A regular sleep schedule is important for the brain.

The key to lasting change is starting small and building on basic victories as we move into 2024. I wish you a healthy New Year!

1. What your body really requires

Everything else aside, there are four things the human body must have to survive: water, food, oxygen, and a functional nervous system.

Humans may endure a little while without food or drink, but life would immediately be over without oxygen or a working neurological system.

What necessities are needed for survival? Shelter, heat, and clothes are likely to be among the top 10. In addition, while these are helpful and will make any scenario more pleasant, they are not needed. At the end of the day, there are just four things a body needs to survive: water, food, oxygen, and a functional nervous system.

Water is more than just a thirst-quencher. Water has a role in nearly all systems in the body, and it is essential to the functioning of almost every system. The human body is around 70% water.

Water regulates body temperature and helps the liver and kidneys flush away impurities. Water lubricates joints and hydrates the eyes, nose, and mouth. Even oxygen and nutrients are transported to cells by water. Without water, the body cannot function.

A person in a variety of ways, including through breathing, sweating, and even going to the bathroom, can lose water. To maintain a healthy body, people need to refill water levels and continue drinking water throughout the day.

Direct water consumption is optimal. Beverages such as electrolyte drinks and fruit such as watermelon can help replace the body's water supply. The standard advice is that women drink a minimum of 11.5 glasses of water every day and men 15.5 cups.

Food offers the body the necessary nutrients. These nutrients are in turn required for energy, cell growth, and repair. Food keeps the immune system happy, and, as a result, poor diets often lead to multiple health problems.

Food can be broken down into four essential groups: fats, carbs, protein, and vitamins. Fats offer energy and help absorb vitamins. Fats can lower cholesterol levels and are needed for growth and development. Carbohydrates are transformed into fuel.

Fiber is a type of food that assists in digestion, maintains blood sugar levels, and keeps hunger levels in line. Protein helps the body restore damaged organs, tissues, and bones.

Protein is contained in every cell in the human body. The digestive tract breaks down proteins into amino acids. There are 20 amino acids the body requires to function properly.

And while the body can make 12, there are still 8 that must be ingested through diet. Vitamins play a part in every biological function. The human body needs 13 types of vitamins to function correctly. Oxygen is breath.

Everything else is spared; without oxygen, life is not possible. Oxygen is breathed into the lungs and then disseminated throughout the body by red blood cells.

Oxygen delivers energy to cells by burning through the sugar and fatty acids that are eaten. In addition to transporting oxygen throughout the body, red blood cells are also responsible for transporting carbon dioxide from the body. Exhaling also removes carbon dioxide from the body.

The nervous system is the body's command center. Information is gathered by the nervous system, which then processes what it gathers and reacts appropriately. The system controls movement by sending nerve impulses between the brain and the rest of the body. The messages move through neurons, synapses, and neurotransmitters. These messages tell the heart to beat, the lungs to breathe, and the limbs to move. Even the way the brain thinks is controlled by the nervous system in general.

The nervous system includes two parts: the central and peripheral. The spinal cord and brain constitute the nervous system at the center. The peripheral nervous system makes up the rest of the body.

Chapter 5

How a full body reset can help fight sickness and preserve your life throughout.

Basic healthy practices are related to living a longer life. If, at age 50, you've never smoked, maintain a healthy weight, are routinely active, follow a nutritious diet, and restrict alcohol to moderate consumption, you could live up to 14 years longer. Making even a couple of these adjustments could increase your lifespan.

Healthy practices can minimize the risk of different diseases, including those that may run in your family. For example, in a recent study, people who followed a conventional American diet (high in fruits and vegetables) for 8 weeks had a lower risk of cardiovascular disease.

In another 2020 study source, researchers discovered that every 66-gram increase in daily fruit and vegetable intake was connected with a 25 percent decreased chance of acquiring type 2 diabetes. Swapping out some refined carbohydrates for whole grains also lessens the risk of disease.

In an observational, reliable study of approximately 200,000 adults, those who ate the most whole grains had a 29 percent reduced rate of type 2 diabetes compared to those who ate the least.

A review of 45 reliable sources of research indicated that eating 90 grams (or three 30-gram portions) of whole grains daily lowered the risk of cardiovascular disease by 22 percent, coronary heart disease by 19 percent, and cancer by 15 percent.

You can extend your life by years with just 11 minutes of exercise per day. In a 2020 study, researchers tracked more than 44,000 people.

Those who got 11 minutes of moderate-to-vigorous physical activity each day had a decreased risk of death compared to those who only exercised at the same intensity for 2 minutes. This comparison held true even if they sat for 8.5 hours per day.

A healthy lifestyle cannot only help you feel better, but it can also reduce the risk of several diseases, lengthen your lifetime, save you money, and improve the environment. Your concept of a healthy lifestyle is whatever you define it to be.

There is nothing you must or must not do to be healthy. Identify what makes you feel good and what provides you with the greatest happiness. Then, start small when you make improvements. You are more likely to see success this way, and minor successes will snowball into bigger rewards.

Lastly, if you want support with making any lifestyle changes, go to your doctor. If they cannot directly help you, they may recommend other professionals, such as licensed dietitians or therapists.

1. You will save money too.

It is always smart to see your primary care physician for an annual physical exam. This is especially true considering how some health issues, such as high blood pressure, are "silent." This implies they do not have any symptoms; thus, until you are tested, you usually do not know you have the problem.

However, the healthier you are, the less likely you will be to see a doctor. This could save money by decreasing co-pays and the need for medicines and other treatments.

2. How an entire body reset can help keep your mind sharp

Some forgetfulness, like occasionally forgetting to pay a payment or recollecting a word, can be expected at any age. But cognitive impairment, such as frequently failing to recall monthly bills or stay focused in discussions, is not a natural aspect of becoming older, according to the National Institute on Aging.

The truth is, your mind, like your physical body, is always capable of change, for better or for worse. In addition, the degree and nature of that change have less to do with age and more to do with action.

It is commonly recognized that if you work out consistently, you can boost your body's performance. For instance, with the correct training regimen, you can enhance how quickly you run a mile or increase the amount of weight you can lift.

However, if you do not exercise and spend hours sitting each day, it will lead to linked bad health implications, such as a higher risk of stroke, research has indicated.

What many people do not realize is that, just like your body, the performance of your mind improves with good and continuous exercise. Likewise, when not provided adequate input, your brain becomes less capable of achieving ideal levels and more sensitive to decline.

You have the power to train your mind for greater sharpness and help shield it from degeneration in the future. Read on for five science-proven tactics you can start utilizing today to create a stronger brain that will serve you well into your golden years.

These tactics are based on the "five pillars for brain health," as defined in CNN Chief Medical Correspondent "Keep Sharp: Build a Better Brain at Any Age," written by Dr. Sanjay Gupta.

(a) Stretch your mind.

The saying "use it or lose it" applies to both your body and brain. Keeping your brain sharp involves keeping it actively occupied. In his book, Gupta alludes to a French study of nearly half a million people, indicating that those who retired at age 65 had a 15% reduced risk of acquiring dementia compared to those who retired five years earlier.

Research also suggests that the quality of brain engagement is important for increasing brain resilience over the long term. That means taking it a step further than the sheer recall needs of a crossword puzzle and engaging in activities that require logic, problem-solving, and obtaining new knowledge.

If you have always desired to study another language, this is a terrific incentive. Consider attempting something new with an online cooking class, starting a new hobby, or reading a nonfiction book that is outside your realm of competence. You may also wish to try internet-brain games that involve quick thinking.

Unlike puzzles that simply help with working memory, speed-processing games have been demonstrated to lessen the chance of acquiring dementia.

(b) Rest your body and brain.

Sleep is not just a time of rest but also a crucial repair process that affects all systems of the body. This is especially true for the brain, which needs quality, deep sleep nightly for memory consolidation.

The US Centers for Disease Control and Prevention states that 1 in 3 Americans do not receive the necessary seven or more hours of sleep per night.

The good news is that getting the regular daily activity indicated above for greater brain health will help you sleep better. Because deep breathing helps you utilize your parasympathetic "rest-and-restore" part of your nervous system, you can leverage your breathing to help you sleep. Another crucial part of relaxing your brain is giving it regular pauses from stress.

This is crucial for brain health, as a high level of the stress hormone cortisol is connected to brain inflammation, cognitive loss, and a higher risk of Alzheimer's disease.

Thankfully, exercise is an effective stress reliever. Other research-backed stress-relieving exercises include meditation, deep breathing, and mind-body practices like yoga and tai chi.

(c) Connect with others

Over the years, various studies have proven that good social ties contribute to better and happier lives. But, when it comes to brain health, current studies have revealed that interactions also boost neuroplasticity, the brain's ability to change, enhance, and preserve its cognitive capacities.

Human beings are social animals; thus, it is not surprising those relationships play a role in brain health. It is crucial to actively cultivate existing relationships through frequent communication and foster new ones by taking part in new activities.

You can quadruple your brain-boosting benefits by socializing in an exercise class or joining a reading club or interest group.

Finally, you should feel empowered to take responsibility for your brain health, starting today. Taking proactive steps to increase your brain's health and performance will serve you for many years to come.

CONCLUSION

The Body Reset Diet, created by celebrity trainer Harley Pasternak, is a 15-day smoothie-focused program that focuses on low-intensity activity. It was popular after Jessica Simpson claimed she had shed 100 pounds in six months.

The diet dispels the myth that slowing metabolisms and weight gain are inevitable and offers a motivational explanation of age-related changes in our bodies. It does not use diet phases, meal windows, or calorie restriction. The Complete Body Reset was developed by the American Association of Retired Persons (AARP) and approved by an international board.

It includes six simple secrets and recipes for real-world use and a dining guide for compliance in popular restaurants. The diet is effective and easy to follow.

The Body Reset Diet is a three-phase plan consisting of smoothies, snacks, and solid meals. Phase 1 replaces breakfast, lunch, and dinner with smoothies, with two snacks per day.

Phase 2 replaces two meals with smoothies, one full dinner, and two snacks daily. Phase 3 replaces one meal with a smoothie, two reduced-calorie meals, and two snacks daily.

After 15 days, there are no formal endpoints for weight loss or maintenance, but the routine and habits acquired are to be followed for a lifetime.

A diet and fitness routine can help you optimize your genetically shaped body. By working out and eating healthily, you can lose weight, increase muscle mass, and feel more energetic. Reshaping your body composition can enhance stamina and make you look firmer.

The amount of reshaping depends on your current physique, time commitment, and dedication.

Before starting a diet and fitness plan, identify your desired reshaping goals. The amount of reshaping depends on your current body type and lifestyle. For example, reducing body fat to a healthy 18% or 25% can be feasible for overweight individuals.

A new year is a time for making health-related changes, but many people forget their resolutions due to their lofty goals. To establish lasting changes, make them simple and make small changes. Here are six strategies for better health:

1. Reduce salt intake by consuming whole foods and plant-based foods, making more food at home, and avoiding prepared goods and fast food.

2. Lose weight by reducing calories and eating complete foods and plants. Start by walking small distances and gradually increase your activity.

3. Partner with your primary care physician to understand your health history and screening needs.

4. Be smoke-free, as smoking is the largest cause of preventable mortality and disease. Consider calling the New York State Smokers' Quitline for help.

5. Reduce stress by identifying problem areas and making time for self-care, such as meditation or using mobile apps.

6. Ensure adequate sleep, as it helps with learning, memory, stress relief, and weight gain.

For adults, aim for seven to nine hours of sleep, while kids and teens need more.

The human body requires four essential necessities for survival: water, food, oxygen, and a functional nervous system. Water is essential for regulating body temperature, flushing impurities, lubricating joints, and transporting oxygen and nutrients to cells.

It is essential for maintaining a healthy body, and direct water consumption is recommended. Food provides the necessary nutrients for energy, cell growth, and repair, and it keeps the immune system happy. It can be divided into four essential groups: fats, carbohydrates, protein, and vitamins.

Fats provide energy, carbohydrates provide fuel, fiber aids digestion, and protein helps restore damaged organs, tissues, and bones. Vitamins play a crucial role in every biological function. Oxygen is vital for life, as it is breathed into the lungs and disseminated throughout the body by red blood cells.

The nervous system controls movement by sending nerve impulses between the brain and the rest of the body, directing the heart, lungs, and limbs to move. The central nervous system consists of the brain and spinal cord, while the peripheral nervous system comprises the rest of the body.

Maintaining a healthy lifestyle can lead to a longer life, with studies showing that a healthy weight, regular exercise, a nutritious diet, and moderate alcohol consumption can increase lifespan by up to 14 years. Healthy practices can also reduce the risk of various diseases, including those that may run in the family.

For instance, a conventional American diet high in fruits and vegetables can lower the risk of cardiovascular disease and type 2 diabetes. Whole grains, such as 90 grams daily, can lower the risk of cardiovascular disease, coronary heart disease, and cancer. Exercise, even for 11 minutes a day, can reduce the risk of death. A healthy lifestyle is personal and can lead to significant benefits.